Fitness for Women

Butt Workout Done Easy

Jordan Miller

Legal & disclaimer

The concept and ideas expressed in this book are purely intended for educational purposes and should not be taken to substitute any form of medical, legal or professional advice.

The author and publisher of this book have provided accurate and reliable material to the best of their knowledge. The publisher is not obligated to provide the reader with additional services such as accounting services or any other kind of service. It is the readers' responsibility to consult the necessary qualified personnel on the specific field the reader has interest in.

The author and publisher of this book cannot be held accountable for any injury, damage or

Dedication

When it comes to who this book series should be dedicated to a lot of names pop up. First of all, I want to think mum for being mum. Mum always believed I would eventually succeed no matter how many times I failed. I would like to think dad for helping me with a place to live when I had fallen on my face. I thank all of my followers that have supported me through the bright and dark. I would like to thank my friend Jason Bracht and Scott Jay for personally helping me with this journey. More than anything I dedicate this book to every women out there who may be misinformed about fitness and training, who may be lost when it comes to making curvy gains, and who just need that extra push to achieve her goals. May I also thank my friend Kendall, it was our conversation that initially seeded the idea of this book series. I would like to thank all of the people who have inspired me personally on YouTube and Instagram.

Table of contents

Preface

Before you read this book and this series I want you to understand why I wrote it.

Around the beginning of 2016, near the end of January, I had been receiving a lot of questions about how to build the butt.

Naturally being an online fitness coach I answered as many of the questions as possible.

Common questions

1. How can I get a booty?

2. What exercises should I do?

3. What do you think of the 30-day fitness challenges?

4. What should I do in the gym every day?

5. How many days a week should I workout?

Now, these are not all of the questions I receive, but they are the most commonly asked questions.

Common concerns

1. I don't want to get overly muscular

2. I don't want people to stare at me

3. I don't have that much time.

One night near the end of January 2016 I was texting a friend of mine. She was asking me what she could do to get the booty, and I came back with the sarcastic response "I should just write a book about it." She agreed that writing a booty book would be a good idea, and then I answered a couple of her questions. The ironic thing was that the whole booty book thing was a big joke. I felt like I was becoming overwhelmed with the same questions and there was not enough of me to go around and answer them all.

1 Week later...

One week after the initial joke of an idea I decided to do some research. It turned out there weren't any decent quality fitness books specifically for booty building. I did find one book that looked nice but had irrelevant content.

It was a bit odd to me that there weren't any genuinely helpful booty building books out there. At first, I wondered if there was no market for booty building short books. After thinking it over I realized my clients were the market; the market was right in front of my eyes. This validated that I could reach out and help thousands of women this way.

Why short books work

Have you ever tried to read a 400-page book about fitness? No? Me neither. Fiction books over 100 pages are great, you can get lost in them, and you can become completely immersed in the drama. You would be lucky to get through 10 pages of most fitness books before falling asleep. When you're reading non-fiction, especially fitness content, less is more. If you're looking for a giant fitness book that you can brag to your friends about completing, this is not the one. Some of the most powerful books ever written are less than 100 pages. The value of a book shouldn't be based off of the amount of volume, but by the quantity of value per page. I am going to make a bold statement here and say my little book will provide you more value on sub 100 pages then some fitness books do in 200 pages.

Let's change things

I believe one big reason there is not much content out there on fitness for women is because most of you are afraid of fitness. You're scared of being judged, afraid of being masculine, and worried about becoming too big. I am here to change that, there is no reason to be scared who you can become. You are going to become sexy and strong.

Disclaimer

Please review the following User Agreement carefully before using the exercises in this book.

I strongly recommend that you consult with your physician before beginning any exercise program.

You should be in good physical condition and be able to participate any of the exercises mentioned in this book.

I am not a licensed medical care provider and represent that I have no expertise in diagnosing, examining, or treating medical conditions of any kind, or in determining the effect of any specific exercise on a medical condition.

You should understand that when participating in any exercise or exercise program, there is the possibility of physical injury. If you engage in any exercise in this book, you agree that you do so at your own risk, are voluntarily participating in these activities, assume all risk of injury to yourself, and agree to release and discharge me the writer from any and all claims or causes of action, known or unknown, arising.

INTRODUCTION

Building a lifted, big, curvy booty has always been an attractive part of the female fitness industry. Guys want abs, and girls want the booty. This isn't just part of the fitness industry anymore, it's quickly becoming a popular part of modern body culture. With this popularity comes a lot of questions, and a lot of unqualified people attempting to answer them. One of my personal favorite trends is the 30-day squat challenge, or even the 60 or 90, your ass isn't going to look like the picture that you're buying into after some bodyweight squats. Many girls are afraid of weights, because they see guys lifting weights and becoming bulky. Random home workouts aren't going to help you, you won't build an ass from a squat challenge made by a marketer with no fitness experience, and you're not going to get bulky by putting some weight on your back. I am going to completely open your eyes in less than an hour. I'm going to break through all of your limiting beliefs about building the booty, as well as shine the light on some marketing gimmicks and BS about building your butt. After reading this book of booty building knowledge you will understand why some things work to build the glute muscle, and why some things are much less efficient. You will learn how progressive overload works, and all the different ways to make those cheeky gains, also the correct form, and what does what. You will, in fact, be able to turn around and educate your best friend on how to also build the booty. You will probably post pictures on Instagram of the booty, because why not you built it with a book the cost of a Starbucks coffee. Ironically, now you can use your butt as a coffee holder. Pat yourself on the back you've just discovered the key to building the booty you want!

Chapter 1: Dispelling the Booty BS

Lifting Weights will make you Bulky

"If you use weights you're going to look like a big bulky man."

The notion that lifting weights makes you bulky is simply not true. Lifting weights, or squatting with weights like a barbell, EZ curl bar, or dumbbells is not going to make you bulky. Without weights, you won't get very far in the progression of having a nice built butt. Everyone has a certain set of genetics, some people are bulky by nature, and some people are more petite by nature. What you can't do is change your genetics, what you can do is shape your body by building muscle. The butt is made up of three muscles, gluteus maximus, gluteus medius, and gluteus minimus. The gluteus muscles need to be broken down so that they can rebuild themselves bigger and stronger. To get results, you're going to need to utilize weight training.

30, 60, 90 Day Squat Challenge

You may be able to see a slightly noticeable difference in a 30-day squat challenge if you don't stand up much, and literally never squat down to pick anything up. However, if you are physical at all, you're not going to make much progress doing these bodyweights squats. I'm not saying bodyweight squats are bad, or that squat challenges are bad. Think about this, whenever you do a leg workout with weights at the gym and the workout has some real intensity to it you probably won't be able to do it again tomorrow. In one intense gym leg workout, you will build more muscle than you would in an entire week of your little squat challenge. If you really want an ass to be proud of, put some weight on your back and drop that ass. Just sitting in the comfort of your little home dwelling doing bodyweight squats isn't going to help you build a booty.

Lifting Super Light Weights makes you Toned

Light weight is a step above being scared of weights, and a step above the thirty-day squat challenge. Now you understand that weights are needed to break down the muscle, so where do we go from here? First of all, I don't want you to be afraid of lifting some decent weight, to break down the muscle you have to exhaust it, this means using more than 5-pound dumbbells. My recommendation, stick between 5-15 repetitions. Going too high in reps isn't really going to create the tear in the muscle you need to induce hypertrophy, which is the growth of muscle tissue. If you go too low in reps you aren't really building much muscle either, you're working your CNS (central nervous system) which means you are getting stronger but not developing an ass. If you're an absolute beginner, it is a much better idea to start at the higher end of the spectrum as far as reps, 10-12 is a great place to start. By beginning with a moderately high rep range, you won't become overwhelmed and you will be able to learn correct form without killing yourself. Eventually, you will find what works best for you. It's critical to choose a weight that will challenge you every single set. If you're squatting with 45 pounds on your back for 12 reps, and you have 12 reps left in the tank you're not going to induce hypertrophy of the cheeky muscles. You need to choose a weight that challenges your mind and body on every set without sacrificing form. You should be hitting 80-90 percent of your maximum effort. Shoot for 1-2 reps left in the tank per set, each set matching the last.

Whether you have 3, 4, or 5 sets, by the last couple of sets you should be leaning towards 90% effort.

You can't workout everyday

There is no certain amount of days you can or can't workout. The frequency in which you exercise depends on three things, your overall workout volume per day, your intensity, and your workload. Let's look at the 30-day booty building super ultra-butt workout plan. Since you're doing a bodyweight squat and you're only doing one set of how many ever reps that day calls for, your volume is low, your intensity is low, and your workload is your own body. This is why you can do it every day, seven days a week, for a month. To be completely honest, if you can work the same muscle every day you're not doing very much. On the contrary, if you go to the gym and do 10 sets of 10 on squats at 99% of your bodies capability of completing each set, followed by 10 sets of leg press at the same intensity doing 12 reps per set, then you walk over to the glute machine and grind out 5 sets of isolated glute presses for 12 reps per set, then you end your workout with walking lunges 5 sets 15 reps, you can't do it tomorrow. Now that was a very extreme, if you did that much volume with 99% intensity, and high workload you wouldn't want to move for 3 days or be able to work the booty again for at least 3-4 days. One of the best places to start regarding butt workout frequency is 3 times per week with moderate volume, that way you're not killing yourself, but you are doing enough to make gains and you can do it again every couple of days!

Chapter 2: The Truth about Building the Booty

Progressive Overload

The gradual increase of stress placed upon the body during exercise training.

Pay close attention to this chapter, progressive overload is the basis of building muscle, especially glutes. The great thing is you can use this info to build any muscle, I am giving you the blueprint to build muscle!

There are three main forms of progressive overload and many other forms that are commonly overlooked.

- Increase weight
- Increase reps
- Increase volume
- Perfect form
- Increase range of motion
- Decrease rest time between sets
- Increase intensity
- Increase frequency
- Adding relative strength
- Tempo

Increase Weight & Reps

If you walked into a gym and asked a random gym guy how to build muscle, what do you think he would probably say? The classic thing to say is, well just lift more weight and do more reps, that's what you're new gym friend would tell you. These are the two most common forms of progressive overload that most people know about. If you were to start out squatting with the 45-pound bar for 3 sets of 10 the first week, that's 45x3x10, weight times sets times reps. The progression would look something like this week; 1 45x3x10, week 2 50x3x9, week 3 55x3x8, week 4 60x3x7. This is a fundamental progressive overload based off increasing weight, the problem here is that you can only gain 5 pound on a lift for so many weeks. After you have been lifting for a while, it will be 5 pounds a month, 5 pounds every 2-3 months, and eventually 5 pounds every year. Another fundamental progressive overload tool is increasing reps. Same idea except you're not changing the weight; week 1 45x3x10, week 2 45x3x11, week 3 45x3x12, week 4 45x3x13. Now you have 2 different variables to play around with. Contrary to popular believe no 1 progressive overload tool trumps all others, but adding weight to the bar, and reps to your sets is most popular. Trying to hit progression in multiple areas every week can lead you very quickly to a plateau, so work smarter not harder. As long as you're progressing you will be making booty gains!

Increase Volume & Frequency

Volume is one of the most powerful tools in your arsenal when it comes to progressive overload. There are a couple of different form of volume, first is your volume per exercise which is going to be your total reps and sets at a particular weight, the simplest way to increase volume this way is to increase the amount of sets you are doing every week. For example, let's go back to the same squat numbers as we previously discussed 45x3x10 would be week 1, week 2 would be 45x4x9, week 3 would be 45x5x8, week 4 45x6x7; That would be increasing volume per exercise, you can also increase your overall volume for the entire workout. When you are increasing your total workout volume, it could simply be you adding a new exercise to your butt workout, or it could mean adding an extra set to one of the exercises, or if you're feeling like taking a beating, adding a set to multiple exercises. Volume isn't just sets its everything. Volume is weight times sets, times reps; however the easiest way to gain the most volume the fastest is by adding on sets to your lifts. I am giving you the tools you need to sculpt, shape, and build the muscle. Frequency is another form of volume, just on a larger scale. To put it simply as an example, if you did squats 45x3x10 once per week, adding frequency would be to add this lift to another day of your week. So, week 1 squats on Monday 45x3x10, week 2 squats on Monday and Wednesday 45x3x10, week 3 and 4 repeat, week 5 and 6 squats Monday, Wednesday, and Friday 45x3x10. Hopefully, you're starting to understand that building an ass actually does take some work on your part. But let me tell you, making progress every week is a beautiful thing; that's why people don't stop working out once they have started. Progress is addictive.

Increase Range of Motion & and Perfecting Form

When you walk into the gym, there always seems to be that guy doing quarter squats with much more weight than he can handle. If you can't squat with a weight to a 90-degree angle or bellow, that is too much weight for you. Before you do anything else make sure you're exercising using a full range of motion, with correct form. For example, when squatting you want to be sure to have your feet aligned with one another as if you're standing on a line; keep straight, chest up, hips back, and keep your back and core tight never letting your back round out, and as that ass drops into your decent breath in; on your way back up blow out! One other thing- rest the bar on your upper trap muscle, shoulder level. Please do not place the bar at the base of your neck as this could result in spinal injury. Excellent form means no injury, and it also means better booty gains.

Focusing on Tempo & Decreasing Rest Time between Sets

Let's talk about tempo, and time under tension! Tempo is the rate or speed of motion or activity, pace of the lift. Time under tension is the total amount of time spent on one single repetition, and also, the time spent on the whole set. Tempo and time under tension are two forms of progressive overload that are widely overlooked by most gym goers. There are three different parts of any exercise: concentric, isometric, and eccentric. The time you take to make it through each portion of the rep can be changed to your liking. Let's break this down using squats as an example yet again. The eccentric part of the movement is the negative part of the rep; this is going from a standing position into the squat. Then you have the isometric portion which is the meat of the rep; this would be where you have squatted down into the hole. The end of the rep would be your concentric part of the movement. In this part of the movement, you are ascending back up to a standing position. You can slow down each portion of the rep to create progressive overload by having the muscle under tension for longer. You can increase the eccentric part of the movement to two seconds as opposed to the typical half a second descent; this will create a little more time under tension in each rep. Another thing you can do is a pause rep, this means you are pausing in the isometric part of the movement, anywhere from one to three seconds. Pausing will make the rep work you much harder, and you can also slow down your concentric motion which would provide even more of a challenge for your battle cheeks. I would recommend not to go to crazy with the time under tension because it can literally triple the intensity of a set. Start out with just pause reps, or just a slow eccentric motion and then go for more! You want to keep the same tempo throughout the entire set. Focusing in, and dialing in tempo is another great way to progressively overload a muscle. The cleaner your sets are, the more progress you will make. You want every rep of every set to look the same, or as close as possible to each other, consistently practicing great form, great technique, sets and reps that are all in harmony. You can look at a great clean workout just as you would look at a really skilled artist; every single note they hit has a purpose. For you, every single rep has a purpose, to build that booty. Knowing this stuff will have you 10 steps ahead of everyone else trying to build a booty because you will understand what it truly takes, and everyone else will be asking you what you're doing. To complement time under tension, and tempo, you can also change the time you spend between sets; for instance if you take 2 minutes between sets drop it to 1 minute, then work on getting it down to 30 seconds. Rest time will be a unique form of overload that you can utilize at any moment if you're short on time, or if you are working on the efficiency of your workout in general.

Increasing Intensity & adding Relative Strength

Have you ever heard of the term emotional fitness? Maybe you have, maybe you haven't. Basically, what it means is that every day you walk into the gym you have a mission; make me better, make me stronger, make me sexier, and make me elite. Everyone has their reason for coming into the gym, and beginning to build the booty, for you, it's a form of power. Don't just go to the gym to build your ass, go to the gym to build your body, mind and soul. When you put some weight on your back remember why you're doing this, because you are redesigning your sense of self, right here and now. If you are ever angry about anything in life, now is the time to use that energy, now is the time to bring the fire. You may become very well educated on building an ass, and any muscle for that matter by reading this chapter, but if you don't get emotional about getting what you want, knowledge won't get you very far. Don't sit by and passively watch as others succeed; don't dabble- take what is yours! That attitude will ensure that you get results. Trust me, you will do things you never thought possible with the right level of intensity.

Last but not least is relative strength. This basically means where has your strength, reps, volume, form, frequency, time between sets, etc. gone once your bodyweight has raised or dropped. One clear indicator that you have built some solid muscle is if you have progressed in any way or multiple ways of progression, all while losing 5 pounds. Even if you've maintained your current lift stats while losing weight, that is also a sure sign that you are making progress! It's really easy to gain strength while gaining weight, but not so easy to improve when you're losing weight. Your strength and your capacity of workload is relative to your bodyweight, so make sure you take that into account when you're following and documenting your progress.

Chapter 3: 7 Powerful Booty Building Tips

Stretch it out

Stretching may seem like common sense; Common sense is not something we see much of these days. Whether you're doing squats, lunges, or kickbacks stretching beforehand is a must for several reasons. Just like an athlete on the field, you do not want to take use of a muscle that is not yet ready to fire. So before you begin your first exercise get to stretching, make sure to stretch out your quads, calves, butt, lower back, and core. Training a muscle that is not properly stretched is a recipe for disaster, it will cause terrible form, discomfort and aches, and you will be putting yourself in harm's way. On the contrary, the wrong kind of stretching can also hurt you. Make sure you are doing dynamic stretching pre-workout, and not static stretching.

Warm it up

Now that you are stretched out and feeling good you need to warm the muscles up to prime them for load. This is probably the only time bodyweight squats are helpful; you want to concentrate on the fluidity of the movement to get warmed up properly. For example, if you're warming up with a bodyweight squat focus on the eccentric portion of the movement, along with the isometric portion of the movement. Warming up gets the muscles warm and ready for a load, and it gets all of the muscles involved in the squat firing; namely the glute muscles, the hips, hamstrings, and core. When all of your muscles are firing you're ready to make some booty gains!

Yoga

Yoga probably doesn't come to mind when you're thinking about building the booty, but it should, and here's why. We have already talked about stretching before a workout, well yoga can be used as an advanced form of stretching, especially on days you aren't exercising the booty. Doing yoga helps to increase blood flow to the muscle by stretching out the areas that may be beat up from all the work you are putting in at the gym to build your butt. Yoga also helps with muscle recovery. This is because when you're getting increased blood flow to the muscles, this attracts more oxygen to the area helping muscles to heal and grow. Yoga is also very helpful in preventing injuries in your next workout and will help you to be much more effective in your next workout by helping your muscles fire more efficiently. One really neat thing is that it can actually help increase progressive overload on future workouts by increasing your capability for range of motion, in turn, helping you get better reps and form on your exercises.

Butt Targeting Cardio

When you walk on the treadmill, take a mental note of how well your glutes are firing while walking. Don't just simply walk to pass time; with every step make sure to contract your cheeks to incorporate some glute activation into your boring treadmill cardio. Try turning the treadmill to full incline- this will target the butt a little better than flat treadmill walking will. The elliptical can also be an excellent accessory to your glute training; simply focus on contracting that booty on every stroke forward on the elliptical. There is one holy cardio machine that trumps all other cardio machines regarding booty activation, it's called the stair stepper, and it is one of the best pieces of cardio equipment for glute activation.

When on the stair stepper take it slow, don't worry about going fast; we aren't trying to get winded, we are building the booty. With every step contract the muscle and you will be making admirable contributions to your booty gains.

Diet Check

This should be another part of common sense, but that still doesn't take away the fact that you do need to pay attention to what you eat. Make sure that you are consuming a adequate amount of protein so that when you're breaking down the muscles in your booty. Your muscles need protein to rebuild themselves. Shoot for anywhere between .75 to 1.00 grams of protein per pound of bodyweight per day, especially the day of, and after training. Also, make sure to get enough carbs in to fuel your workout, namely fruits and veggies. You need carbs to fuel the muscle; protein may rebuild muscle but that will never happen without carbs. It's not usually too big of an issue to get fats into your diet, especially if you eat out often. However, you do need fats, so don't cut them out. Fats are your slow burning fuels that fuel your mind and body, and regulate bodily functions;

you need them more than you may think you do.

Write it down

Now that you have a keen understanding of how to build the booty through progressive overload, the next best thing you could possibly do is write your workouts down every day. Get yourself a little notebook or diary and write everything down. Write down the exercises, weight, sets, reps, and if you're feeling like a badass take notes on your form, rest between sets, tempo, and time under tension, as well as how you felt that day. This way, every week you can see where progress is being made, and make changes from there, the more info, the better. It's even a great idea to write down your weigh-ins every morning. How far you want to go is completely up to you, everyone has different lifestyles, and everyone has different goals; do what works best for you, and most of all don't take it too seriously. I am giving you a toolbox, but you don't always need to be using every single tool. Sometimes you can't really see or comprehend how much progress you have made and are currently making unless you can physically look at last week, the week before,

3 weeks back, 1 month, 6 months, and 1 year back. Another thing writing your workouts down will do is help you understand your body, and how you personally progress. Everyone's body is a little different; it's important to learn yours.

Forced Reps, Super Sets, and Drop Sets

These are some volume adding techniques to increase intensity, eliminate time between sets, and drop to set after set. Forced reps aren't really something I recommend for beginners, but after a while, they can be a useful tool to progressively overload the booty by forcing in an extra rep or two. Basically, a forced rep is performed by having a spotter assist you in performing one or more reps past your body's point of failure. I don't recommend forced reps often but it can be a nice little overload tool to break through plateaus every once in a while. Super sets are where you have 2 exercises and you're performing them back to back; this can be an excellent way to add some volume to your booty training when you're short of time, or looking to add a little extra volume in an unconventional way. This is also a shortcut to completely eliminating your time between sets. With a drop set, you perform your last set to failure. For example, let's say you're doing 10 reps of lunges with 35-pound dumbbells. Immediately after that set you drop the weight to 20 and perform another 10 reps with lighter weight; followed by that you drop the weight again for a second time and perform another set of 10 reps with 10 pounds dumbbells with even lighter weight and at the end of your nice little drop set you drop the weights and perform 10 reps doing bodyweight lunges. Trust me when I say drop sets are no joke; I recommend you put in some time in the gym before using any of these advanced techniques. But once you feel that you are ready these can be a great additions to your booty gains, I wouldn't do them every workout, just whenever you need them. These are just 3 more weapons to add to your ass building arsenal.

Chapter 4: Get the Booty

Working out and building muscle certainly comes down to a science. There is no question about it; if you follow the advice in this book you will build muscle, you will build a booty. However you can have all of the tools, all of the info, all of the tips, and still not have your mind right. This chapter is all about what's in your head, setting off the fire within, and getting your mind primed to kick some ass literally.

Visualize the Booty

Before you walk into the gym, sit in the car and turn the music up, think about what you're about to do; see it, feel it, and taste it. Get your mind ready for war; war with yourself, war with the weights. You aren't just going into the gym to talk and get a little baby workout in, you're going into the gym to build "That Ass." You have decided that enough is enough- it's time to make some changes, it's time to take control of your life and build the booty you want. What do you want to happen in the gym today, what do you want to accomplish, what do you want to feel, what numbers do you want to hit, what exercises are you going to do? Are you going for a rep PR (personal record) today, are you going to hit a weight PR, set PR, are you going to get your form to the point where your exercises have the tempo of a well-executed dance? What are your goals for the week, what are your goals for the month, the year? Today when you walk into the gym you're moving one step closer to that goal, whether you achieve it or not is on you, so find that fire and turn it up!

10 Reasons for the Booty

The biggest reasons that some people get great results and other people get no results comes down to two things. Are you having to push yourself to do this, or are you being pulled? It's very popular for people to say, just do what you're passionate about, just do what you love and results will come as a bi-product. I'm not saying not to do what you love, but what I am saying is that there is more to it than that. You are either pulled towards sometimes because you have several reasons as to why you are doing it, or are having to push yourself to do something because you aren't sure why you're doing it, just maybe because others are doing it, and it's sexy. To put it simply results are sexy, however, the process is not as sexy, but it can be fun and fulfilling. Ask yourself why do I want to make this happen, what will having a developed ass do for me? I have been working out for almost 10 years; the reason I workout now is because progress is a crucial part of my everyday life, but getting started wasn't so easy. I needed confidence, I needed to love myself more, and I needed to take my mind, soul and body to another level. Whatever interested you in building a booty in the first place, remember that. Do you want an ass that drives people crazy, I know some of you do; write that down. Do you want to build a social media presence and show your progress, maybe you do, write that down too. I am guessing you want to inspire and motivate others with your sexy booty, am I right? Do you want to feel good about yourself, have more confidence, and want respect? Whatever the reasons are as to why you're embarking on this booty build journey, write it down, at least 10 things; the more the better- make it fire.

Hold yourself to it

Sometimes it's easy to say I have done great for the week, I'm going to take my next workout off, and sometimes you truly need a break. However, sometimes you're actually hurting yourself in private. Once you establish with yourself that you can take workouts off you start to adopt the mindset that you need a break here, and you need a break there; this mindset is for weak minded people with terrible work ethics, so stay away from this mentality. Get a workout partner if you know anybody that is also looking to build a booty, and you know they will kick ass with you; ask that person on a gym date. Then ask them to be your gym partner, you hold them accountable, and, in turn, they hold you accountable. You push them, they push you, and a littler friendly competition can be helpful to make those gains as well. Another option to hold yourself accountable and to help push forward is to hire a coach, not a personal trainer, but a coach. What a coach does is hold you to what you're supposed to. Most serious coaches only take on clients that can prove to them that they are serious about making progress. Each week you report to your coach with all of your stats, how your workouts went, you can even report your weigh-ins and what you ate. Your coach will set new targets, and make new goals from there, and it will be up to you to meet these goals, you will be held to it.

Booty Pics

Having a nice booty has always been popular; it's only recently that the booty has become so popular, and even gets you paid sponsorships. This is a product of Instagram, which is a big part of the upward trend of ass pics everywhere. If it doesn't offend you, and it doesn't make you feel butt hurt about your own butt, then it most likely motivates you. Start a fitness oriented Instagram page and use it to document your progress flat to phat, why not? When things work for you share the knowledge, when you're feeling good about your gains post about it. To some this will be narcissistic, especially lazy people with a negative attitude towards fitness and body image. To others it could be that last little bit of fire to get their ass in shape, that may even have been you at some point or you now. Whatever you do, do it for yourself, and for others, your new-found ass can be a weapon of mass destruction or it can be a reminder that if you put in the work, you will look incredibly sexy, and you will feel really good about yourself.

Conclusion

Let me first congratulate you on finding this little booty building book! There are a lot of misinformation out there; as a result of that there are a lot of misinformed people out there. We live in a world where we want everything fast and easy, so that is what everyone markets and sells. I have no idea where the notion that working out with weights makes girls bulky came from, it is simply not true, and I am very glad that you now know this. My theory is that some highly endorsed celebrity, with a glorified celebrity trainer stated somewhere in some article that lifting weight makes females bulky, and it was probably to sell some sort of as seen on a TV home workout product, because home workout products are trending on Google, which again is because of lazy people that won't leave their little comfort zone. Then there are the 30-day squat challenges, which if you don't move around much they may actually make a small difference and lift your butt a little if it is completely flat, the only reason it does anything at all is because your ass is basically asleep, because it gets no action, by doing a couple of bodyweight squats you're waking it up. When you're actually at the gym progressively overloading the muscle you're building a booty that would make a 30-day squat challenge booty cry. You're now on the opposite side of the fence; you're not afraid anymore, you're not scared of getting too many results or working out too hard- you're ready to make some gains, bring the pain you booty building machine! You now understand progressive overload in its many forms, you have all of the tools to not only get you started, but to keep you going. You're about to become the person that people love to hate, and that's ok because that is a sure sign that you're making gains. It's not about what you do, it's about how you do it; whether you're performing squats, walking lunges, leg press, or hip thrusts. It's all about the progressive overload and the mindset you have. You have dispelled all of the booty BS and discovered the truth about that nonsense; you understand progressive overload, and how to break down and rebuild the muscle, and if you made it to the very end of this book I know you are on fire and ready to kick some ass. So now it's up to you. You have everything you need to build a booty; you were smart enough to spend your pocket change to purchase this book, and now it's time to do the work. I want to thank you personally for investing your time in this book, and I promise you, that if you use everything in this book to better yourself, you will indeed get a booty, and much more.

Sincerely, Jordan Miller

Acknowledgments

I would like to acknowledge all of the people and places I go to for fitness inspiration, and to learn personally. So here we go, time to start throwing out names. I want to acknowledge Christian Guzman for being my biggest source of YouTube inspiration. I would also like to recognize all of the others I watch on a weekly basis for inspiration and knowledge. Here are some of those people –Matt Ogus, Jeff Alberts, Nick Wright, Max Chewning, Raymond "The Online Coach" and many more. I would like to give acknowledgments to Nikki Blackketter for being my favorite YouTube channel for women.

About the Author

Hi, I'm Jordan Miller, writer, and publisher of Fitness for Women.

Here's a little about me: I'm an internet entrepreneur, natural bodybuilder, online fitness coach, and writer.

It's you vs. you, if you're here you probably know that already, you're not going to settle for anything less than extraordinary.

I have been training for about nine years and love every second of it.

At 13 years old in middle school I was jumped by 2 bigger kids for one reason, to humiliate me. My right leg twisted awkwardly and I was told I would need a knee replacement by 25 if I could walk on that leg at all. I was out of school for about 3 months bed ridden, nobody liked me, I didn't have many friends, and girls had no interest in me because I was labeled as "Faggot" which is the word kids my age used to alienate other kids that were different. I didn't have any purpose, I couldn't find any reason to be alive other than to play video games. There were two very clear options- kill myself or create a life with meaning. I chose to live! The second my leg healed I was on a mission to validate who I wanted to become, so I stepped into the gym a loser and came out a fighter. As I got more into health and fitness, I started to have a few followers, made friends with people I wanted to be friends with, and got a girlfriend. Just a couple of years following I decided to compete in an OCB Natural Bodybuilding competition at 15 years old, I got into the best shape of my life and became hungry for success. I competed twice more before the age of 17 and placed well. After learning how to manipulate my body for almost 5 years I wanted to help others. For about a year I helped people for free, then started to make a little money on the side while I was helping people. When it all comes down to it, fitness may have saved my life and I owe it to the world to save other lives. Lots of us want to get into great shape, for guys it's getting a nice chest and nice abs, for women it's the beautiful legs and the booty. I completely understand, and even though I am a guy I wanted an ass myself because I believe it looks good in general male or female. I do practice what I preach. Follow me on Instagram for motivation and specific questions. (JORDANFITT_)